Take a Breath

A Transplant Journey

Karen A. Kelly M.D.

Published by Richter Publishing LLC
www.richterpublishing.com

Editors: Mandi Weems, Jenna Rimensnyder, Diana Fisler & Kenny Darling

ISBN:1945812044

ISBN-13:9781945812040

DISCLAIMER

This book is designed to provide information on lung transplants from a caregiver's view only. This information is provided and sold with the knowledge that the publisher and author do not offer any legal or medical advice. In the case of a need for any such expertise consult with the appropriate professional. This book does not contain all information available on the subject. This book has not been created to be specific to any individual people or organizations' situation or needs. Reasonable efforts have been made to make this book as accurate as possible. However, there may be typographical and or content errors. Therefore, this book should serve only as a general guide and not as the ultimate source of subject information. This book contains information that might be dated or erroneous and is intended only to educate and entertain. The author and publisher shall have no liability or responsibility to any person or entity regarding any loss or damage incurred, or alleged to have incurred, directly or indirectly, by the information contained in this book or as a result of anyone acting or failing to act upon the information in this book. You hereby agree never to sue and to hold the author and publisher harmless from any and all claims arising out of the information contained in this book. You hereby agree to be bound by this disclaimer, covenant not to sue and release. In the interest of full disclosure, this book contains affiliate links that might pay the author or publisher a commission upon any purchase from the company. While the author and publisher take no responsibility for any virus or technical issues that could be caused by such links, the business practices of these companies and or the performance of any product or service, the author or publisher has used the product or service and makes a recommendation in good faith based on that experience. This book reflects the author's present recollections of experiences over time. Some names and characteristics have been changed or left out to protect the privacy of individuals. Some events have been compressed, and some dialogue has been recreated. The stories and views in this book are entirely from the author and do not reflect the opinions of the publisher.

DEDICATION

I would like to dedicate this book to my incredibly resilient husband Steve, the generosity of the donor and family, along with the doctors and team at Tampa General Hospital Lung Transplant Program.

CONTENTS

ACKNOWLEDGMENTS

I would like to thank Dr. Melissa Bailey for writing her book, *Pink Hell*, and inviting me to her book gala. At the gala, I won the raffle prize for a book publishing promotion with Tara Richter of Richter Publishing! This event was the true inspiration to begin writing my book. Tara's workshop and books were instrumental. Tara's direction and team of editors and designers have been fantastic.

Steve, thank you for sharing your thoughts and feelings with us about your illness. Your strength, humor and love have been an inspiration to me to tell your story.

I also wish to thank the following people who took their personal time to read, inspire and teach me: Sue LaGree, Dr. Dave and Leslie Weiland, Greg Overcashier, Susan Jenkins, Dr. Anna Sarno, Megan and John Kelly, Adam Magaletta, Pam Ward, Dr. Kim Odom, Dr. Kathy Boreman and Dr. Greg Savel.

FOREWORD

It is often said that *life* is a journey and not just a destination. Occasionally, the ordered ebb and flow of daily life is interrupted by a defining event that is transformative. A serious life threatening illness or untimely death changes, not just the stricken individual, but the social fabric that surrounds them. The impact is not like the ripples in a pond from a cast stone but a seismic shift with permanent change. Every life is uniquely special and interacts with so many others in meaningful ways. Yet these important connections are often obscured by the day to day routine of modern life. This story is one such transformational moment that is unique yet true of many others. Here the patient, loved ones, friends and caregivers are confronted with this threat to life. They first seek answers, then treatments and after miraculous success must ultimately return to daily life under a new paradigm. Truly, the adjustments to the new reality of emotional, financial, and social change can be as difficult as battling the disease itself and require far more patience and endurance. Karen's story is truly inspirational not in just the miracle of organ transplant in modern medicine but the indomitable human spirit that overcomes its side effects.

As a Hospice and Palliative Care specialist and member of a transplant medical review board (MRB) it is important to help families and caregivers to balance the desire for a cure with the sobering realities of the treatment plans. With all the advances in medical science it is important for patients and families to not just focus on the acute treatment of the disease but the impact on the patient and family by the treatment plan. They must be able to cope with healthcare related impact on quality of life lest the clinical success and gift received be lost to despair. Karen and Steve's resilience in this story relate to the strong reliance on humor to cope with the inevitable setbacks. In this case humor is truly the best medicine for coping with the stresses and travails while navigating the rocks and shoals that are frequently encountered in our fragmented healthcare system. It is not enough to endure with the second chance given. We must learn to Live anew to honor the sacrifice of strangers whose lives have intersected with ours.

Written By: *Dr. Dave Weiland M.D.*

INTRODUCTION

Breathing—usually an easy and mindless act. You are doing it now. Take a moment to consciously breathe; feel the air expand your lungs; then exhale and feel the air leave your lungs. Be totally aware of your next breath and take a slow, deep breath in and out. Feel how it relaxes you. Even though this process is vital to our survival, we take this miraculous activity for granted. We may not even realize that we could be holding our breath in excitement or surprise. We may not even feel our breath speeding up during exercise or sighing from sadness, disappointment, or frustration. In order to survive and thrive, we need working lungs. Lungs absorb the oxygen from the surrounding air when we inhale and then release the carbon dioxide from our body when we exhale. We do this an average of 20,000 times every day. Our breathing is regulated involuntarily by our brainstem. This allows our breathing to happen automatically, without us being aware of it.

This book will help you to appreciate every breath of air you take. This is the true story of my husband Steve's journey starting with the destruction of his lungs due to a rapidly progressing irreversible lung disease, through to his miraculous recovery. The life-saving treatment was a lung transplant surgery, along with comprehensive care from a team of physicians and staff at Tampa General Hospital (TGH). This surgery was all possible thanks to another person's ultimate sacrifice of organ donation and untimely death.

Steve at that time was a fifty-five-year-old Irish man from New England who went to trade school and worked as a machinist. I am his wife of twenty-five years, a full-time Tampa Bay pediatrician in a group practice called Myrtle Ave Pediatrics with twenty years of experience. Steve and I met at a health club in Massachusetts playing racquetball before I began medical school in 1989. Steve gave up his career in the machinist industry to stay home and be the primary caretaker raising our children when they were young. He went back to work later in his life as the facilities director for a community health center. We raised two amazingly successful adult children: one graduated from Boston University and is working in her chosen field of film/TV production in New York City; the other is in college studying biology and computer science.

Steve had been the strong, but light-hearted pillar, who supported us through all my years of medical training. My medical training in pediatrics consisted of four additional years in medical school at the University of Massachusetts in Worcester, with three more years in residency specializing in pediatrics. We married during my third year of medical school. We moved to sunny Florida in 1991 so I could do my pediatric residency at All Children's Hospital in St Petersburg, FL. We have always lived an active lifestyle, worked full time, and enjoyed vacations and boating with the family.

When both children left the home in 2013, we were excited to enter this "empty nest" phase of our lives. However, Steve's sudden symptoms of his disease began and we were thrust into a remarkable battle for his life. He was admitted to TGH on the brink of death before the transplant and endured many setbacks. Along every fighting step there were many possibilities for diversions that surely could have resulted in his immediate death. He at times felt that he may not live through the process but he continued to hold onto a positive attitude. His life-changing journey is truly fascinating and exciting. It can resonate with all and teach many lessons along the way.

Throughout the process of Steve's diagnosis and lung transplant, our relationship assumed a new depth and closeness. My role changed from medical practitioner to primary caretaker which allowed me the opportunity to view the other side of patient care. Together we fought through this horrible disease and extensive recovery process. It was difficult to watch my husband go through such pain and suffering. Steve was always so brave and independent when it came to his care and meds. He had incredible strength and resilience with a positive attitude towards recovery. This attitude clearly mattered for Steve in fighting for his life and is truly beneficial for anyone battling a disease.

With the combination of our situation, and my medical training and experience, I offer a unique perspective and advice on this entire journey. The story will provide you with a first-hand look and a better understanding of the complex but fascinating process of receiving a lung transplant. You can read the thoughts and reflections of my husband as he experiences such a serious illness and recovery. You will gain insights and tools to help navigate through the "medical maze". This maze we all inevitably experience as either patients or caregivers within the health care system.

As I watched a second person that I love rapidly deteriorate from the effects of a destructive lung disease, it is a powerful reminder of the utter importance and need for survival that our lungs serve. Ironically, I also cared for my mother who tragically died in 2001 at the age of sixty-one from a devastating lung disease, pulmonary sarcoidosis. She struggled for many years with shortness of breath and was on oxygen through a nasal cannula. At that time the miracle of lung transplant was not readily available.

Presently in the United States there are more than 120,000 people on organ transplant lists. Each day an average of over seventy-five people receive an organ transplant. However mostly due to the shortage of organs, over twenty patients die each day waiting for transplants. The need is real. Please register to be an organ donor at donatelife.net or organdonor.gov.

One strong piece of advice to deal with medical situations is not to be afraid to speak up, ask questions, and listen. If you don't understand what the medical practitioners are saying, or if something doesn't make sense, a simple question could make a major difference in the diagnosis and treatment of the patient. Work as a team with your medical professionals. Ask what to expect and speak up if you or your loved one are not responding to the treatment. You are the one at home able to monitor the patient 24/7, they are not. Advocate for your loved ones by feeling confident enough to ask questions and become informed—no matter what disease you are battling.

As a caregiver, you must also take care of your own needs. Get rest, eat properly, take time to exercise, and take a break from the situation. Along life's journey, especially while navigating the medical process, take moments to be aware of your breathing. Stop, take deep breaths, and relax to appreciate your own working lungs. These meditative moments will calm your body and mind. As a result, you will have more energy to be present in order to help yourself and others.

Finally, I encourage you to incorporate laughter into this process. Laughter is one of the best prescriptions that will help to not only lighten your load, but also that of the patient, caregivers, and medical staff.

Take a Breath

CHAPTER 1: THE BREATHING REQUIREMENT

We really started to take notice of Steve's breathing in September of 2013. We were at parent's weekend at our son John's college, Stetson University. Steve was always in good physical shape. He measured six feet two inches tall and weighed over 200 pounds. During this trip, something odd about Steve started to present itself to me—the long walk from the front desk to the elevator caused him to be short of breath. I noticed he kept stopping to catch his breath. He looked like he had just run a marathon and appeared to be using his extra "accessory" muscles in his neck, back, and abdomen to take deep fast breaths.

Before I go any further, let's take a short detour to explain the breathing requirement so you'll understand this problem better. Breathing is the action of inhaling and exhaling. We contract our diaphragm and chest muscles to expand our lungs to inhale outside air through the mouth. Simply put, take a deep breath right now. As you do this, you will notice your shoulders begin to rise and your ribcage lift. Your stomach will expand slightly as your chest cavity makes room for your lungs to inflate fully with fresh air. This air travels down our windpipe to the bronchial tubes where it reaches small thin sacs, called alveoli. Alveoli are used by our lungs to exchange oxygen (O_2) into the blood for carbon dioxide (CO_2). Think of alveoli as very thin barricades that gases like O_2 and CO_2 can penetrate.

Small blood vessels or capillaries take this oxygen-rich blood to the pulmonary veins which go to the heart to distribute blood to the rest of the body. This oxygenated blood is necessary for every cell and organ in our body to function. Damage can occur to our lungs and body when we continuously breathe in polluted air or cigarette smoke both directly and indirectly from secondhand smoke.

Simultaneously, our body tissues dispose of CO_2 in the blood, which flows to the heart and small vessels leading to the alveoli in the lungs to release. When we exhale, we relax our diaphragm and chest muscles to release CO_2 out our nose and mouth. Exhaling requires no effort at all from our bodies—unless we are exercising or have lung disease. Under these conditions, we need more air so we use those accessory muscles found in the neck, back, and abdomen to assist the diaphragm and chest muscles to help us breathe faster and deeper. That's what

Steve appeared to be doing during this easy stroll down the hallway in the hotel. He was recruiting extra muscles and energy to return his breath back to a normal level.

With all this in mind as I continued to watch him struggle to catch his breath, I was quite surprised, and my first reaction was to blurt out: "What is wrong with you? How long have you been feeling this way?" His response was, "I don't know, maybe for a few months now, but I just thought I was getting older and out of shape from sitting at my desk more at work."

As I watched him walk, I began to worry about many medical conditions. At the top of my list was something wrong with his heart—which could lead to fluid in his lungs and make him short of breath. His father had suffered a heart attack in his fifties. So this put him at higher risk due to his family history of heart disease.

Many times when people are suffering from the progression of lung disease, they don't even notice until their condition has progressed too far. So it takes a family member or friend to notice and push them to seek medical attention. I was quite concerned and made him promise to go to the doctor after the weekend.

Steve had already noticed his shortness of breath was getting worse, which he gauged during his daily walk to and from the parking lot at work. Over weeks he went from being out of breath after the walk to having to stop during the same walk to catch his breath. He realized that he had a problem at that point but was limiting his activity and parking closer to shorten his walk in order to cope. He continued to tell himself he was just out of shape.

Although he had mentioned this to me, I had not witnessed the severity of his breathing until that weekend.

I was reminded of Steve's last experience with a serious medical condition. About eight years earlier, he had been feeling some pain, numbness and tingling in his neck and arm for a while without telling anyone. Finally, he went to have it checked out, and they determined that he needed immediate repair to his cervical discs in the neck area. The surgeon noted that most people with his symptoms seek medical care long before he did. He explained that any sudden jolting of his neck could have resulted in a serious neck injury, even paralysis. He needed surgery urgently, but Steve was not really convinced, and the doctor had to call me to make sure that the surgery was set up immediately.

Steve had barely even mentioned to me that he was having symptoms. Ironically, even though Steve married a doctor, he wasn't too keen on going to the doctor himself, unless he was near death. As we all have experienced, spouses often do not listen to their loved ones about their health, even if their spouse is a doctor. That's why we all have to nag them until they give in and see our way. However, he did admit that he was *thinking* about going to the doctor. In the case of his shortness of breath, he made the appointment right away after that hotel weekend.

He decided to go to one of the internal medicine doctors at the health center where he worked. Surprisingly, his chest sounded normal during the exam.

They ordered tests to take a look at his lungs. The regular chest x-ray was not that abnormal looking. However, the cat scan (CT) of his chest was quite alarming.

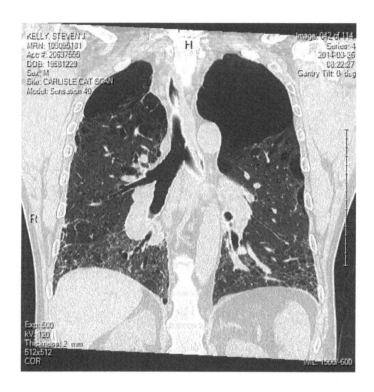

CT scans are a more sophisticated and powerful x-ray machine that takes 360-degree pictures of internal organs. It showed multiple large bubbles, called bullae, in the upper-mid and top parts of both lungs. These were essentially huge open holes in his chest area that should have been filled with lung tissue. These huge areas of his lungs were not doing the job of exchanging gases like they should. The only area with regular working lung tissue was in the lower mid-section. No wonder he couldn't breathe! On the radiology report there was a one-line note of mild pulmonary fibrosis at the bases.

We were referred to a pulmonologist who reviewed the CT scan with us. He was quite impressed by the large bullae. By the way, it is not a good thing when a specialist says "impressive" to your CT! My husband is the king of practical jokes and witty "one liners". He always finds humor in every situation. He soon had the doctor joking with him about how they could drive a truck through the impressively large holes in his lungs.

At this point, everyone was so impressed by the size of these large holes that no one thought twice about the small amount of pulmonary fibrosis at the bases of his lungs on the CT report. It was noted as an afterthought on the CT scan results. They did breathing tests on him called spirometry and other lab tests. Based on all the data, he was given the diagnosis of chronic obstructive pulmonary disease (COPD) or bullous emphysema. This chronic lung disease adversely affects the lungs by creating bubbles—or bullae—which make it hard to get air out of the lungs and breathe. It is commonly caused from exposure to toxic gases, like cigarette smoke and is the third leading cause of death in the United States.

I must take a short digression to inform you about the dangers of secondhand smoke from cigarettes. Secondhand smoke kills more than fifty thousand adults and children every year. That's more deaths than car accidents, alcohol, homicides, suicides, guns, and cocaine combined. Hard to believe isn't it? There is no risk-free level of secondhand smoke. Even brief exposure can have detrimental health effects to vital parts of your body. Your lungs are being damaged just by walking through cigarette smoke outside a doorway, in a car, or in your workplace. Exposure to secondhand smoke can lead to or trigger an asthma attack and other respiratory diseases like COPD and lung cancer. Protect your precious lungs and avoid that cigarette smoke like you would run from someone waving a gun.

Steve was diagnosed with COPD which is an emphysema like disease; therefore he was placed on inhalers to treat this condition. On the first day after the breathing treatment, he felt better. As a result, he was encouraged that his condition was a treatable disease like asthma. He was confident that he would get through this and adjust to life using inhalers from now on. We both researched the disease to become informed. Steve was doing what the literature suggested and attempting to exercise by taking walks around the block to help slowly build up his lungs. During those walks he was extremely short of breath and would have to stop many times to catch his breath by the side of the road. It looked so difficult for him that people would stop to ask him if he was ok.

A few months later, in February, 2014, Steve and I went to a comedy show. During the show we realized that he could hardly laugh or even walk to the car without looking like he had run a marathon. He had to stop and take deep breaths just to get to the car. His disease was getting worse by the week. Steve was feeling the rapid decline in his breathing capacity, and he was losing confidence in his ability to recover. Every day he hoped he would wake up and feel better. He was sure that he couldn't get any worse. It was alarming to watch my strong husband put his head down and take five to ten minutes to calm his breathing rate down to a normal level. I thought he was going to have a heart attack at any moment.

Soon after seeing the pulmonologist for the first time, he developed pneumonia. He recovered from this set back after being treated with antibiotics and steroids. While already in a weakened state, pneumonia could have put him in the hospital and damaged his lungs more—or even killed him. His breathing health continued to decline at a rapid pace. Our friend, an internist, suggested he be placed on oxygen at night. At first he was embarrassed to wear the oxygen in a public place, but soon his condition required him to wear it continuously both day and night.

Each time he had to explain his condition to others was a reality check for him. It was as if his life was changing forever and this was what his "normal" would turn out to be. Still, despite feeling extremely tired and taking frequent naps to regain his energy, he was still confident that he would get through this and be cured of his illness altogether.

This rapid progression did not appear to fit the typical picture of COPD at all. COPD is usually a slowly progressing disease that older people get from smoking. Steve was younger than the target age group, and a non-smoker, yet his difficulty breathing was escalating very quickly. The doctor kept changing the types of breathing treatments, but there was no improvement. Steve, alarmingly, felt himself decline daily. We went back to the pulmonary doctor earlier than suggested.

The doctor was also puzzled by Steve's even further rapid decline of lung function; therefore he was referred for a second opinion to Tampa General Hospital's lung transplant center. TGH is nationally recognized as one of the nation's top hospitals for pulmonology and one of the few hospitals in the state of Florida that perform lung transplants. At that time, in order to be evaluated by a doctor at TGH's lung transplant program, you had to fill out the paperwork and meet certain criteria. As a result of his initial diagnosis of COPD and other pulmonary tests, he surprisingly *did not* meet the criteria. It was unclear as to why he was not classified as severe enough to warrant evaluation for lung transplant because people with COPD can also be candidates for transplant. So we were stuck.

His doctor devised a back-up plan with a referral to another team of specialists in TGH's interventional radiology program. These doctors specialize in performing cutting edge minimally invasive procedures to diagnose and treat many diseases. They were evaluating him for a brand new procedure for COPD in order to essentially vent or pop the large bullae and make room for his good lung tissue to expand and work. They proposed to do one lung in order to save the other side for possible lung transplant in the future. We later were told that this option to pop the bullae would most likely have been devastating to Steve's condition.

Before we scheduled that procedure, we were fortunate enough to have one of the transplant pulmonologists at TGH look at his CT scan—even though Steve did not meet the standard criteria. After reviewing the scan, the doctor called us to come in for an evaluation. They watched Steve walk in the door with his oxygen and immediately determined that he was not suffering from COPD. It turns out the disease causing all the damage was that little footnote of pulmonary fibrosis at the bottom of his lungs. The large holes in the top were something that is not usually seen in this disease, and thus it threw off the doctors in making his diagnosis. However, in Steve's case, those large holes, or bullae, were actually holding room in his lung cavity to be able to accept a larger set of lungs. Thank God for those large bullae. The cause of those bullae was and still is unknown.

REVIEW

1. Properly functioning lungs are a requirement to live. Protect them by avoiding damaging gases like polluted air and cigarette smoke, including secondhand smoke.

2. Exhaling requires no effort at all, unless you are exercising or you have lung disease. Therefore, pay attention to you, or your loved ones. If they are always short of breath or wheezing and coughing with activity, seek medical help.

3.   Ask questions, research, and learn about the disease that you or your loved ones are diagnosed with. Always return to the doctor to seek help or be evaluated if the condition is worsening.

Take a Breath

CHAPTER 2: IRREVERSIBLE LUNG DISEASE: IDIOPATHIC PULMONARY FIBROSIS

The team at TGH diagnosed Steve with idiopathic pulmonary fibrosis (IPF) in May of 2014. Steve's symptoms fit like puzzle pieces into the diagnosis of IPF. We were relieved at first. Steve also tried to throw in some humor by saying, well, at least it isn't cancer. But the Doctor said this condition is worse than cancer! There is no known cure.

Pulmonary fibrosis is a disease in which the lungs become a thick and stiff, "cement-like" material. They become scarred and start to shrink. As the lungs thicken, they cannot properly move oxygen into the blood stream, so organs, like the brain, are deprived of oxygen. Naturally, we asked what caused this disease. In medicine, idiopathic generally means that they don't know the cause. The life expectancy after diagnosis of IPF without treatment is three to five years. Patients die of respiratory failure, heart failure, pulmonary hypertension, pulmonary embolism, pneumonia, and lung cancer.

There is no known cure for IPF and the treatment is a lung transplant. That statement hit us like a brick. Steve felt numb. Hearing those words, he finally understood the seriousness of his condition. In his mind, the next step was simple: do whatever it takes to get the transplant. Our feelings of relief were quickly replaced with fear of what that treatment would entail.

Surprisingly sometimes doctors don't always know the actual cause of diseases nor how people may acquire them. People ask that question all the time at my office. With something like the common cold, we know it is transmitted from droplets spread from sneezing, coughing, or touching. However, we don't know for sure who gave it to you. For Steve's condition, it's possible that something like his past job as a machinist may have exposed him to unusual metals, like beryllium, in the air that could have deposited in his lungs.

For this reason, it is important to wear gear to protect your breathing when you deal with metals and chemicals that become airborne. They hypothesized that beryllium could have laid dormant in his lungs for years. An unknown mechanism triggered the lung cells to react to the metal, leading to the development of this disease. The end result, IPF, caused the cells of his lungs to stop properly exchanging gases. As this disease progressed and the destruction of his lungs became more significant, it became harder to release oxygen into the blood stream.

Due to his body's normal response to try and get more oxygen from the lungs into the blood stream, this constant "stress-state" his body was under led to pulmonary high blood pressure. This in turn led to pulmonary hypertension (PHT)—the narrowed, blocked, or destroyed pathways made it harder for blood to flow and raised the pressure within the lungs. Steve was having unusual symptoms including restless sleep and nightmares. He had a spell where he forgot about his condition, stood up quickly, and then immediately passed out. One time he was at the doctor's office coughing up mucous to give a specimen and he also passed out. All these symptoms are thought to be caused by PHT.

They told us that the large bullae, or holes, were not commonly seen in IPF. His pulmonologist at TGH also stressed that if he would have gone through with the radiological procedure of releasing the bullae in his lungs, it would have likely allowed the fibrosis at the bottom of his lungs to take over what little remaining good lung tissue Steve had left. The bullae were literally acting like a levy to keep down the fibrosis from overtaking all of Steve's lung tissue. With no defenses remaining on his healthy portion of lung, it's almost absolutely certain his symptoms would have worsened even quicker.

During the course of Steve's deterioration, we had opportunities for travel by plane. Everyone seemed to think that it would be okay for him to fly with his condition on oxygen. But when we booked a flight, his instinct told him not to go. Sadly, he wasn't able to travel and see our daughter Megan graduate from Boston University in May of 2014. Of course he was there in spirit and on Facetime! This gut instinct, it turns out, was life saving for him. His pulmonologist at TGH later stressed that changes in pressure would negatively affect his health. In airplanes, the altitude change causes tremendous air pressure differences. This sudden change in pressure to Steve's lungs would have likely popped those bullae leading to breathing decompensation or even death on the plane.

Note to self: when something doesn't feel right, don't force it. Listen to your instincts.

Once Steve was diagnosed with this non-curable lung disease at the first visit, many things began to happen. The impact of a lung transplant on a patient's life is complicated and all-encompassing. In order to help with the stress of this impact, TGH transplant team's overall philosophy was to look at the patient from a holistic approach: medical, social, and financial. Primarily, the diagnosis and medical condition were the foremost criteria to be considered for lung transplant. However, the social and financial aspects were also addressed. These three areas needed to be satisfactory in order to be accepted for transplant. If issues or problems are identified, then measures would be taken to support or rectify them, if possible. They made it clear from the start that getting a lung transplant requires a social network and team of family and friends to support him. The financial burdens are astronomical and they even suggested holding a fundraiser to help. Their goal was to extend his life as long as possible. They want to transplant patients at the right time, not too early and not too late.

The transplant surgery leaves the patient with a lifetime of taking complex medications and a lot of stress from the demands of constant medical treatment and follow-up. Patients must be committed to doing what is necessary to stay healthy. The doctor asked Steve if he was willing to accept these conditions and even give up beer! Of course, he made a joke about that and said, "Well, maybe...".

His doctor was very careful to watch Steve walk and measure his oxygen with a pulse oximeter. This is a small, lighted instrument that goes on the finger and reads the amount of oxygen in the blood. They wanted him to stay between 88-100%. They adjusted Steve's oxygen tank to two liters per minute in order to keep him at that level. They stressed how important oxygen was to keep his heart, kidney, brain, and all other organs from suffering damage.

Next, the transplant team set us up to meet the finance coordinator. He asked us if we had transplant insurance. Who would ever think to ask about that when they get health insurance? Fortunately, when they checked with our insurance, we had transplant coverage, and Tampa General was the preferred hospital! Wow, that was a major stroke of luck. For people who do not have transplant coverage, they suggest methods for fundraising. The average cost from start to finish for a transplant, including all the medicines and procedures, is in the two-million-dollar range. Holy cow! That's enough to make anyone lose their breath!

Next, we met with the pre-transplant coordinator/ nurse. She handed us a list of things we needed to complete before Steve would even be considered a candidate for the transplant list. This list was like a medical scavenger hunt consisting of tests and doctor visits that absolutely must be completed and checked off in order to move forward. This list included visits and notes from a dermatologist, ophthalmologist, gastroenterologist, and dentist that said he had no evidence of cancer, infection, or other medical problems. During the next few weeks he was scheduled for three days of tests and visits at TGH, including a visit with a hospital psychologist to make sure Steve was mentally up for the challenge. Now it was my turn to tease him saying, "Oh no! How will you ever pass a psych test!" Lastly, to make sure his heart was strong enough for this procedure, he also went through a cardiac catheterization.

Along the way, Steve met other patients going through this testing process. On the first day of testing he met two men that appeared to be at least ten years older than him. He started to feel that he was rather young to be going through this disease. These men had their diseases for years and had been to other hospitals but did not make the transplant list. He did not know what exact disease they were diagnosed with, and he felt uncomfortable asking them. One man told him that he had paid twenty thousand dollars to go through a stem cell transplant that did not fix his medical problem. A stem cell transplant is a treatment where the patient's blood is taken out, filtered, and returned intravenously. The theory is that these filtered basic stem cells will deposit in the lungs and begin to rejuvenate new lung tissue. This method is controversial and not effective for many patients. Steve will always remember the look of desperation on this man's face when he pleaded, "Hey you got to try anything!"

He realized that these men were desperately trying to get on the transplant list to save their own lives. Some did not pass the tests and were not able to be considered for transplant. Other patients were able to fix the issues that led to failed tests and reapply. Talking to these patients was scary and discouraging for Steve. At first he thought because he was younger and in better shape, he would surely make the list. He was nervous that if he failed the tests he would need to have a back-up plan. This, and the fact that he was on O2 and in a wheelchair, at times ate away at his confidence to get on the list. He felt it was unfair that these men were each in need of a lung transplant but were being turned away. He had mixed feelings because he did understand that there were only a limited number of lungs available for transplant, and that patients needed to be healthy enough to survive the surgery and extensive recovery.

Finally over a month later, after all his tests and evaluations were completed and he met satisfactory standards, Steve's case was presented to the Medical Review Board (MRB) at TGH. The board consists of:

pulmonologists, surgeons, cardiologists, a social worker, a financial coordinator, and transplant coordinators. This board collaborated to decide whether a single or double lung transplant would be needed, based on their interpretration of his diagnosis and test results. Once accepted, everything is sent to the insurance company for review. The three outcomes from the MRB are either accepted, tabled for issues to be resolved, or rejected.

REVIEW

1. Lung transplant is a treatment for idiopathic pulmonary fibrosis (IPF), which is an irreversible lung disease. Other diseases that may lead to lung transplant are severe COPD, cystic fibrosis, and idiopathic pulmonary hypertension.

2. Listen to your instincts when it comes to your health, if it doesn't feel right, don't force it.

3. When you get health insurance, look into all of the coverages, including transplant. **PLEASE consider a donation to non-profit funds to help transplant patients like Lifelink Legacy Fund.**

4. Wear recommended gear to protect your precious lungs when you deal with airborne chemicals and avoid pollution and secondhand smoke.

Take a Breath

CHAPTER 3: THE WAITING LIST

In July 2014, we got a call from the transplant nurse coordinator. She informed us that Steve was accepted for the transplant list! Before Steve could be officially placed on the waiting list, we had to go through a mandatory listing talk that was specific for the waiting patient and their immediate caregivers. During this two-hour meeting, they took him into another room and gave him vaccinations against diseases, including pneumonia, hepatitis, tetanus, and pertussis. This is done as an important preventative precaution. Once Steve gets the transplant, he cannot fight off infections well due to the required medicines that will suppress his immune system.

They also met with Steve's mandatory care team, which consisted of close family and friends. On that day, at the end of the meeting, Steve was officially placed on the list. We were required to be on-call 24/7. We had to be ready to drop everything and rush to TGH within an hour's time. They encourage each family member to always have a phone on and charged, dependable transportation, and be ready to leave at a moment's notice. Steve needed to have a personal bag packed and ready to take to the hospital. In preparation for his surgery, the coordinator required one of us to schedule being with Steve 24/7 for three months following the transplant.

They explained to us that the waiting list is overseen by the United Network of Organ Sharing (UNOS). UNOS, a non-profit charitable organization, manages the nation's transplant system, known as the Organ Procurement and Transplantation Network (OPTN). These programs are under contract with the federal government. UNOS and OPTN operate by dividing states into eleven regions with each having separate lists. Florida is in Region 3, as shown in the chart below (lung.txp.com):

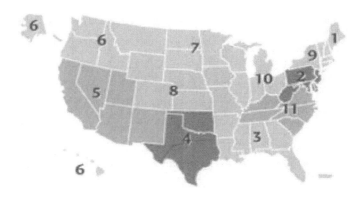

All regions have different Organ Procurement Organizations (OPO). There are 58 OPO in the United States. The one for our section of Region 3 is LifeLink.

To find the one for your region go to organdonor.gov.

LifeLink has a coordinator who stays in constant contact with the transplant coordinators. They inform the transplant coordinators of possible donors, and the transplant coordinators inform them of possible recipients.

At first, patients on the waiting list like Steve will be listed according to their blood type. Due to the different blood types and antigens, donors must be compatible with different recipient types. For instance:

☐ Donor with Blood Type **O** can donate to **A, B, AB & O**

☐ Donor with Blood Type **A** can donate to **A & AB**

☐ Donor with Blood Type **B** can donate to **B & AB**

☐ Donor with Blood Type **AB** can donate to **AB** only. (lung.txp.com)

Different heights must be compatible as well. For height, a donor can be up to twelve inches taller or eight inches shorter than the recipient. The heights need to be compatible in order for the donor's lungs to fit into the chest cavity of the recipient.

So they called Steve a "tall A" meaning he is tall and has the blood type A. This is encouraging because recipients with blood type A can get a donor with either blood type O or A, which happen to be common. The absolute best blood type to have as a recipient is AB, because they can accept the blood type of any donor.

The next criterion is called the lung allocation score (LAS), which is an individualized number between 1 and 100. This number will determine a recipient's priority on the waiting list. It is assigned by a complicated calculation that basically predicts how long a patient is likely to live without a lung transplant and how long a patient would be expected to live after receiving a lung transplant.

Steve's LAS was 65, which was determined to be moderately high—the higher the number, the higher the priority, and thus the higher a recipient is placed on the waiting list. This LAS number is calculated using many factors related to the patient's condition. Some of these factors include a patient's diagnosis, age, oxygen requirement, blood chemistries, and body mass index. Medical researchers designed this LAS by studying scientific data on lung transplantation with different lung diseases. Steve's doctor stressed how important it was to let them know immediately of any changes in his condition, because this could significantly change his LAS.

According to the scientific registry of transplant, there were between forty to fifty patients on the lung transplant list at TGH during the year, June 2014-2015. For the entire United States, 1,700 people were listed on the lung transplant registry for that period. During the year of 2014, it is noted that 29,532 people in the U.S. actually received organ transplants. At any one time there are an average of 120,000 people in the U.S. on transplant waiting lists for all organs. Those lists are constantly changing as people receive their transplants or are taken off the list. Presently each day in the U.S. an average of over 70 patients receive an organ transplant. However over 20 patients each day die before receiving one mostly because of the shortage of organs. (organdonor.gov) Please register to be a donor at donatelife.net.

For many people, depending on their condition, this waiting list can last for months—or even years. As you can imagine, this can make life very complicated. At the beginning, people on the list are fully prepared and ready to go. After years of patiently waiting on the list, that mindset can begin to contrast with itself. Months, which can turn into years, make it hard to keep your whole life confined to within an hour's distance from the hospital. Patients can temporarily take themselves off the list while traveling away from the hospital. Patients with a slower disease like COPD commonly wait a long time on the transplant list because their condition is usually not as critical, so they are lower on the list.

When the time for transplant comes, there are usually two types of calls. The first call is, "We have an offer of lungs for you so please come to the hospital immediately. Do not eat or drink anything." Or the second call is, "We have an offer of lungs for someone else but due to special circumstances, we need to bring you in as a back-up. So come to TGH as soon as possible." Both patients will be prepared for surgery, including receiving meds such as antibiotics, steroids, and immunosuppressants to prepare them for transplant. These meds are not harmful to the patient even if they don't receive the lungs.

As Steve and I digested all this information at the end

of this two-hour meeting with his care team, he was placed moderately high on the transplant list. We then went home to wait for the call. Steve was able to work part-time from home doing computer work and phone consults. At home, he passed the time resting and taking frequent naps. He had limited energy to do any physical labor around the house. This was frustrating for him because he always had projects going on at home. Steve was able to joke about it and say, "Hey, I feel like I'm living the retired life, just like your dad!"

Obviously, there was no way to predict when a set of lungs for Steve would become available. We were waiting for someone in Region 3 with the correct blood type and size to tragically die and become a donor. Many people wait for extended periods of time. For Steve, after he was already on the transplant list for two weeks, his oxygen requirements began to rise slowly over the course of a couple of days. That is, to maintain his pulse oximeter above 88%, it became necessary for Steve to increase his oxygen flow through the nasal cannula. This was reason enough to call the transplant nurse and report his changes.

Steve was a little hesitant to call immediately. When he finally did call the transplant nurse, they asked him to report to clinic promptly to be evaluated. He stubbornly insisted on driving himself to the clinic in Tampa. He technically was not breaking any rules as long as he remained on his O2 tank continuously, he felt completely fine to drive. Most of all, he did not want to be a bother to anyone. His independent personality found it so hard to ask for help or depend on anyone else. This attitude can be such an asset for survival, but dealing with it can surely be a curse. At times I wanted to strangle him over it. Once he was seen in the clinic, the transplant pulmonary doctor sternly scolded him for not calling sooner. At that point, they determined he was too sick to go home, and admitted him to TGH.

That first night in the hospital was frightening because the medical staff kept having to increase Steve's oxygen levels. The levels were going higher and higher, and I wondered what happened when they reached the top amount of oxygen. He ended up on thirty liters of heated high-flow oxygen administered through a funny looking large tube to his nose (see picture at end of book). Remember, he began with needing only two liters of oxygen, and now he was on thirty.   That amount of oxygen can only be delivered in the hospital, and it severely dries out the nose. In order to make it tolerable, the doctors had to use heated humidified air. Now Steve was told, "You are staying in the hospital until you get the transplant."

I was horrified by his rapid decline, and felt badly for him being so debilitated. I was extremely thankful, however, that he made it onto the transplant list before his lung function rapidly deteriorated. At the same time, I was so mad at Steve for not letting someone drive him to the hospital, but ultimately I could not fault him for being independent and maintaining a determined attitude about the whole situation. Mostly, I was relieved that he was going to stay in the hospital so he could be monitored. I jokingly asked the doctors and nurses, if it wasn't too much trouble, could they throw in a personality transplant too. That gave everyone a good laugh and lightened the entire situation.

Even though his lung disease had taken a turn for the worse, Steve was still feeling fine while he sat at rest in the hospital on high levels of oxygen. He was even able to do some work on his laptop from the bed. But as soon as he would get up to go to the bathroom, or walk around the bed, his oxygen levels would drop. They hooked him up to even more oxygen for the few minutes that he needed when he went in the bathroom and when the physical therapists took him for a walk for his therapy. They jokingly called this oxygen apparatus the "twin turbos'". His lungs at that point were totally destroyed by the disease with only a small working section left to function for basic breathing.

At first after he was admitted, Steve felt confident in the doctors and the hospital and believed that he would be fine. He felt that he would just get new lungs and go on with his normal life. However, as days passed in the hospital, he suffered bouts of feeling depressed, thinking his life was over and that this was it—no more wife, kids, or friends. His recurring thought was that he just wanted to go home, have a cold beer, and forget about everything.

Due to this rapid deterioration, leading to hospitalization and an increased oxygen requirement, Steve's lung allocation number was increased significantly. This increase catapulted him to the top of the transplant waiting list for all of Region 3. The hospital staff also told us that if a matched donor became available outside of our region, due to his serious condition, they would notify us for a possible match. Steve was extremely critical and placed at one of the rarely seen highest positions on the transplant list. This reality slap got Steve to joke about his new life or death scenario by saying, "I'm either going home with new lungs or new wings".

Thank goodness the method of placing people on the transplant list had changed. In the past patients received transplants on a first come first serve basis. Due to the scarcity of lung donors, many patients would die before ever getting a lung transplant. Lungs are very fragile compared to other organs. The protocol, by following the LAS, effectively uses the limited number of donor lungs available and as a result has reduced the number of deaths among people waiting for a lung transplant.

REVIEW

1. It is a difficult task, like performing a medical scavenger hunt, to pass all the tests needed to get on the lung transplant list. Many patients don't make it. Once you make it on the list, you go home to wait for a donor.

2. Donors and recipients for lungs are effectively matched by region, blood type, size, and then severity of illness.

3. The new protocol for using the limited amount of available lung transplants has worked well to reduce the amount of deaths among people on the waiting list.

3. In the U.S., there were an average of 120,000 people on organ transplant waiting lists. 1,700 of those were for lung transplants during the time when Steve was on the list (June 2014-2015). However, largely due to the shortage of donors, each day over 20 patients die waiting. **PLEASE register to be a donor at donatelife.net or organdonor.gov.**

Karen A. Kelly M.D.

CHAPTER 4: ULTIMATE SACRIFICE

Organ donation is a gift that provides renewed life to a patient in critical need. After a life-saving heart, liver, lung, kidney, pancreas, or small intestine transplant, many recipients go on to lead normal, active, and productive lives. A single donor could save eight lives, and impact dozens more through tissue donation. Annually 28,000 transplants are made possible by donors. The need for donors is real because over twenty patients a day die waiting for organ donors. Please consider becoming a donor. To register to be a donor visit www.DonateLifeFlorida.org or outside of Florida visit www.DonateLife.net.

How does a person become a donor? Organ donation for large central organs like the heart and lungs usually occurs after someone has suffered an injury that results in brain death. A donor must have sustained some form of head and brain trauma, like a motor vehicle accident or gunshot wound to the head. A stroke, brain aneurysm rupture, or heart attack can also deprive the brain of oxygen. When the brain is deprived of oxygen long enough, it stops working, and has no active cells or neurons to properly function. It essentially dies, and the donor is then pronounced brain dead by stringent medical criteria while the heart is still beating, and the body is maintained on a ventilator. Many people have fears over donating their organs. One fear is that they may be treated differently as a patient. I assure you that your life comes first and doctors work hard to save every person's life. A patient is declared a donor only when there is complete and irreversible loss of brain function.

The LifeLink foundation was established as a non-profit organization with a commitment to saving lives through organ and tissue donation. It was established more than thirty years ago by a nephrologist, Dr. Dana Shires. LifeLink covers the areas of central Florida, Georgia, and Puerto Rico, by linking the transplant recipients with the life-saving organs of donors. LifeLink's Organ Recovery Organizations (OPO) serve as a crucial link between these donors and recipients. LifeLink and the OPO serve 250 hospitals and ten transplant centers while serving a total population of over 16 million people within this designated service area. (LifeLinkfoundation.org) To find the organization for other areas go to organdonor.gov.

LifeLink is notified by the medical staff of this person's potential brain death at any time of day or night. LifeLink then decides if this is a possible transplant donor candidate. If the match is a go, then the message is given to the transplant center associated with the recipient patient who matches the donor. At that time, the surgical team immediately goes to harvest the organs. We were told that because lungs are especially fragile, there is only a 50% chance that the team will be able to harvest those lungs. So once you get the call that there is a matched donor, there is only a one in two chance that those lungs will be used for the transplant.

Steve had been sitting in a hospital bed at TGH waiting for someone in our region to die a horrible death. Either this person would already have to be registered as a donor or their family would have to be generous enough to say "yes" to an organ donation after suffering this terrible tragedy at the deceased's bedside. Obviously Steve was in dire need of lungs but to be "hoping for someone to die soon" was an unusually mixed sentiment.

Once the donor was accepted, we could not be told who the donor was or where the lungs were coming from. This information is confidential, and that is the protocol. There is a system through LifeLink where the donor's family or the recipient may write a letter. This letter goes through LifeLink for screening. Some families decline to be contacted. This is done at a respectful time later. Steve and our family are extremely thankful for the donor and family's generosity in allowing for organ donation. Our thoughts and prayers go out to wish them peace and comfort. The decision to allow for donation saved Steve's life along with many others.

After a few days in the hospital, we were told a potential donor became available. But once they reviewed the details, the donor was too small. That donor then was passed on to another person on the regional list. Two days later another donor became available, but this one was too big.

Steve was given the nickname "Goldilocks" by the hospital crew. We were hopeful that the next donor available would be just right. He thankfully was not dropping his oxygen levels any more, but his condition was critically in need of a lung transplant. At least he was able to sit in the hospital bed working on his laptop to keep his mind occupied. Family and friends sent him cartoons, jokes and funny pictures to keep him entertained. His mind remained quick witted and his fingers fired back teasing texts as fast as a teenager! I was working my usual hours in my pediatric practice. We were communicating by text, calls, and post-workday visits. He was being safely taken care of in the hospital. Then on August 26th, 2014 at 5:30am, I was doing my hospital rounds seeing babies in the nursery, when Steve texted me that something was up.

REVIEW

1. Organ donation is the ultimate sacrifice and a gift that provides renewed life to critical and dying patients.

2. LifeLink is this region's non-profit organ recovery organization that serves to link donors with recipients.

3. A single donor can save eight lives and many transplant patients go on to lead normal productive lives.

4. To register to be an organ donor go to www.DonateLifeFlorida.org or outside of Florida www.DonateLife.net and sign up.

Karen A. Kelly M.D.

CHAPTER 5: LUNG TRANSPLANT

Steve's medical team canceled his food and started to do some preparations on him. They didn't tell him any details yet because he was already at the hospital, and there is always a 50% chance that the lungs would not be recoverable. Most patients on the transplant list are just being called to the hospital at this point.

Since he was already at the hospital, he texted me a warning to be ready. Of course, as fate would have it, my partners in my pediatric practice were putting their lives on hold to support my efforts with Steve. But when things were dragging a bit, we encouraged my partner to go on a trip to see his daughter in school in New England. Wouldn't you know it, as soon as he got on the plane that day the correct lungs became available.

By the time I got there, around noon, they were prepping Steve for surgery. They cleaned him up with antibacterial washes, put on socks to prevent blood clots, and gave him anti-rejection meds. We were told that the transplant team was on a plane to harvest the lungs. It was still possible that once they inspected the lungs, they could call it off.

Around three o'clock in the afternoon he was wheeled to the pre-op area of the cardio-thoracic transplant operating room (OR), which looked like it was out of a "science-fiction" movie. Then things moved quickly—they called for Steve to go directly to the OR—no time for the holding room. They handed me his wedding ring and we said our goodbyes. This was it. After two and a half weeks of waiting in the hospital, in critical condition at the top of the transplant list, Steve was about to get new lungs...well maybe!

The thought that I may never see him alive again crossed my mind. I felt terrified, but also excited that the time was finally here that could save his life. No one could tell me at that moment what was to come. My heart was racing and I was ready to run a marathon, but instead I was escorted to the surgical waiting room to sit, wait and pray.

Family and close friends joined me for support. There was much nervous energy in that room. We always tried to lighten the mood with jokes. My husband, Goldilocks, had found the perfect or "just right" sized lungs. The surgery began at four in the afternoon. The surgeons worked on one side at a time where they opened Steve up under the ribs (see figure below: lungtxp.com). His ribs were then lifted to perform the surgery.

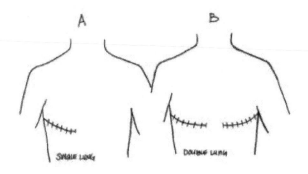

The surgical transplant team put Steve under with general anesthesia and placed him on a cardiopulmonary bypass machine. While on bypass, the blood is pumped and enriched with oxygen by a machine, rather than by the heart and lungs. While they had him on bypass, they did not need to stop his heart. This bypass machine has been used by doctors for years when performing many types of common heart surgeries.

After the team completed one side, they sent a nurse out to say that things were going well. They were listening to music while they worked, "Eye of the Tiger" is what they chose. Finally, the surgeon came out at the end of the ten-hour procedure looking completely exhausted. The surgeon said it was a difficult task getting Steve's diseased lungs out. Due to the scarring on his lungs and adhesions to the side of his chest cavity, a lot of bleeding occurred in the process. I was told that Steve may experience a significant amount of pain while healing, but the lungs the surgeon put in place were pink, beautiful, and fit perfectly. This was truly a miracle.

Next, Steve was monitored in the post-op area,

before being moved to the surgical ICU. The doctors allowed us to see him through the window. No visitors were allowed in the first twenty-four hours due to Steve's critical condition. He appeared pale, swollen, and puffy in his face. There were intravenous (IV) lines from his arms and central lines from his neck. He had chest tubes draining fluid from his surgical area. He also had a tube in his mouth to breathe. He was hooked up to many machines and monitors. I was distressed to see my husband lying there motionless, yet I was elated that the surgery went well.

Steve was heavily sedated at first; then slowly, over twenty-four hours, he was weaned off the sedation meds. This was in preparation for extubation—removing the tube to breathe on his own. I talked to his nurse in the ICU from home that first night. As they lowered his sedation, Steve surprisingly woke up with the breathing tube in place and almost pulled it out not knowing what he was doing. That would have been a disaster because the surgical sutures that attach the new lungs were near the breathing tube. If he pulled out the breathing tube, it would have disrupted the sutures. Thankfully, they were able to give him more sedation to keep him calm. In the past, even when he had minor surgery, he needed extremely large "horse" doses of medicines to knock him out. This was surely a testament to his tough, stubborn Irish heritage. You really can't keep a good "Irish" man down-like it or not!

Steve's many lines and tubes were working to keep him alive. The IV lines in his arms and neck provided him with fluids, meds, and even nutrition for recovery until he could eat on his own. Chest tubes are necessary after chest surgery to help build back the negative pressure in the chest necessary for the lungs to expand. Tubes from the chest are also needed to drain all the fluid and blood from the surgery. In Steve's case, due to all the scarring and adhesions in his chest from his damaged lungs, a lot of blood and fluid continued to drain out of those chest drains for several days after surgery.

Following a transplant, the lungs are stiff and need time to get used to their new "home." Steve still required some oxygen for a few days after the surgery. This is common with lung transplant patients.

Because some nerves attached to the lungs, heart, and diaphragm are cut during the transplant, there are a number of side-effects that follow surgery. Steve didn't feel the urge to cough so they taught him to take deep breaths and cough frequently to clear secretions. He also used an exercise machine for the lungs that he breathed into to help move the secretions and inflate his lungs. His heart rate didn't respond as fast to exertion because of the cut nerves. Some patients may notice a change in their voice from healing and possible damage to the nerves of the vocal cords. This, thankfully, did not happen to Steve. So he could continue to tease me and others with his deep, booming voice!

Steve spent five days in the ICU after the surgery. Before they could let him eat or drink anything by mouth, he had to pass a swallow test. This was to ensure that he could swallow both liquids and solids without aspirating into the new lungs. The lungs are also at risk for damage from acid indigestion. So patients are treated with antacid meds to prevent this condition from damaging the new lungs.

We learned a corny hospital joke from the nurses: Why do they make you wear those gowns in the hospital that keep on opening up to show all your private parts? Because you're in the 'I See You' (ICU). The nurses are true compassionate heroes in the hospital. We are particularly thankful for all the attentive care given by the nurses and supporting staff along every step of Steve's journey.

Steve was extremely thirsty when he woke up in the ICU. This is a normal reaction for the body to experience when it hasn't had fluids by mouth. They had only been giving him IV fluids. Oddly, he asked for grapefruit juice as his first post-op drink. However, there are specific guidelines for transplant patients regarding their dietary restrictions. They had given us the list of foods while he was in the hospital. One of the forbidden drinks is grapefruit juice because it interacts with the transplant medicines. Here I was ready to get him anything he wanted post-op, but when he asked me for that, I just looked at him stunned and said, "What? You can't have that, Honey."

We're not sure why that request came out first; he had never liked grapefruit juice before. It could have been because he had read about it before the surgery in the booklet, prompting his mind to think of it after. Or perhaps it was just because he HATES to be told what he can and cannot do! Either way, he first passed the test to drink a thickened fluid like apple juice or lemonade. Steve complained it tasted awful and had a weird consistency...just like my cooking!

Steve's physical recovery began next as the therapist got him up to sit in the chair and even stand. He could hardly put weight on his legs. It was surprising to see how weak this big, strong guy was after the surgery. He was beginning the long road to recovery.

Visitors were always required to wear mask, gloves, and gowns to protect him from germs. After passing his swallow tests, getting his central line and some of the drains out, he was moved to the transplant floor. This is a big day. They called it his birthday or "rebirth" on the transplant floor. They even got him a "Congratulations" cake. Celebrating each small milestone is an excellent way to focus on the positive and further aid the healing process.

Every transplant patient is placed on multiple meds post-operatively. Pain meds at first are needed to help recover from the major surgery. Sometimes laxatives and stool softeners are needed to balance the constipation side-effects common with pain meds.

Most importantly anti-rejection meds are given to suppress the immune system. These crucial meds help stop the body from rejecting the transplanted organ. Steve's body will always view these lungs as foreign tissue and will always try to reject them. As an unwanted side effect to these necessary meds, his immune system cannot fight off any type of infection as well. Steve was also placed on antibiotics, antiviral, and anti-fungal meds to protect him from every form of infection. Post-op anti-clotting meds and heart meds are also standard and were necessary to help regulate his body after the surgery.

After a few days on the transplant floor, Steve developed an irregular fast heart rate called atrial fibrillation (AFib). His blood pressure dropped and he became unstable. He was immediately transferred back to the ICU for monitoring. They called me soon after I had returned home from visiting him. As I walked into the ICU, I expected to see him in a bad state, but he just smiled and said, "Don't eat the fish." The doctors and staff had a nice laugh! They were all surprised that he looked that alert and awake in the ICU with AFib.

Heart problems can be commonly seen after transplant surgery, because some of the nerves to the heart are cut during the surgery. It is amazing to think that you can survive and do well without those nerves. In Steve's case, they had to switch the cardiac med because that first one did not agree with his heart rhythm. His heart rate stabilized on a different med, and he was transferred back to the transplant floor after twenty-four hours.

Steve felt his recovery was rough. His thoughts were that he had no oxygen, and despite the medical people saying he was doing great, he felt like "crap" and he had lost a lot of weight. His attitude remained positive and he continued to be an excellent patient. Steve thought, "If they say I am doing good then I will keep on fighting." Soon after, his recovery became smoother sailing. He spent one more week in the hospital.

These final days on the hospital transplant floor were filled with activities intended to help ensure his long-term success, including physical therapy and rehabilitation exercises that made him strong enough to go home with a walker. Steve along with family members of his care team received educational sessions from pharmacy, nutrition, therapists, and the nurse transplant coordinator to learn all the complicated lifelong meds, diet, and health-monitoring plans necessary for survival.

For the discharge planning, the transplant nurse coordinator surprisingly told us, "You owe us a rejection and an infection." That meant that these problems are actually expected and can be easily treated if caught early. However, they are usually fatal if not treated or are discovered later in the process. The nurse instructed Steve to take all of his meds. To stress her point, she told us how some young adult patients (usually with Cystic Fibrosis) feel so fantastic after having a lung transplant that they decide not to take their meds—then they die. It was shocking to hear this, but it was necessary to warn us not to ever take recovery for granted.

Finally, we heard the words, "It's time to go home." We could hardly believe it. At this point, Steve had been in the cocoon of the hospital for over a month. He spent two weeks before his transplant waiting for the lungs, then recovered after the transplant for another two weeks. The average hospital stay after lung transplant is one to three weeks. He had dropped fifty pounds and had a full beard. He was at his high school weight and looked like a different person.

REVIEW

1. Lungs are so fragile that 50% of the time the donor lungs cannot be used for transplant. Lung transplant surgery is commonly performed with an under the rib approach, general anesthesia, and cardiac bypass. Patients commonly stay 1-3 weeks post-transplant in the hospital.

2. To ensure long-term survival after transplant, patients and their care team receive extensive instructions from pharmacists, nutritionists, therapists, and the nurse transplant coordinator to learn all the complicated life-long meds, diet and health-monitoring protocols.

3. Rejection and infection of the transplanted lungs are so common that they expect it, and are treatable if caught early.

Take a Breath

CHAPTER 6: FINALLY BACK HOME...
NOT FOR LONG

On a Friday afternoon, September 2014, I drove the forty-five minutes from Tampa to Dunedin with Steve in the passenger seat. He was nervous to leave the cocoon of the hospital. He felt he needed to go home, but he was not feeling ready to deal with life at home. I was certainly nervous to have him home, but tried not to show it. He wore a mask and gloves to protect him from infection. Amazingly, he was wearing no oxygen. On the drive home I cringed as I watched him painfully feel every bump in the road. When we pulled in the garage, he needed help to get out with a walker. He sat in his favorite chair in the kitchen and was relieved and happy to be home. Our cat, Pippa, was delighted to see him. The rules following a transplant do allow interaction with dogs and cats, but recipients are not allowed to handle feces and precautions must be taken to avoid scratches or bites. Absolutely no litter box cleaning due to the bacterial spores thrown from the cat litter into the air. Best excuse ever to get out of that chore, don't you agree?

Steve slept well in his bed the first night. It was much more peaceful than the hospital, where he was woken up every few hours with tests and vitals. Ironically, you never really rest in a hospital.

There are some specific nutritional guidelines for post-transplant patients that must be followed, including no blue cheese, raw meat, fish, and eggs due to the fungus and bacteria these foods might harbor. It is also important to wash every vegetable and fruit with mild soap and water. Due to his excessive weight loss, it was vital for Steve to have healthy and well-balanced meals—specifically extra protein to help him build his strength back up. Our family and friends were eager to support his recovery. Many of them offered us gifts of food to help. During those first few weeks, soups were his favorite food to feast on. They were easy to eat and provided good nutrition.

On his first morning home, Steve requested peanut butter toast for breakfast. Within thirty minutes of eating breakfast, he started to feel short of breath. His oxygen level was dropping, as measured by the pulse oximeter. We had oxygen at the house from before the transplant, and we placed him on it. We called the transplant center. On the phone, the transplant nurse questioned whether the pulse oximeter read correctly on Steve. Sometimes it takes adjusting to get it to read properly. However, he really looked like he was having a hard time breathing, and we kept having to increase the oxygen levels. He started to gasp for air and looked at me with wide eyes. I immediately called 911. I was terrified that something had gone terribly wrong.

As instructed by the transplant team, I told the firefighters and paramedics that since he was a newly transplanted patient, they could not pick him up under his arms because it would pull on the surgery site. They could not press on his chest to perform CPR because of the surgery. They also could not intubate him or put a tube into his trachea to help him breath because it could disrupt the internal surgical site where the lungs were attached. The firefighters were ingenious. They grabbed Steve's home office wheelie desk chair and propped him in that to take him out to the ambulance bed. Steve will always remember fading in and out of consciousness in that ambulance, and hearing the paramedic scream, "Get me the bag!" His only thought was, "This can't be it? All I have been through and I only made it home for one day." They were able to get a mask over his mouth and nose (bipap) to provide him with enough oxygen pressure to keep him comfortable during transport to the hospital. Like nurses, paramedics and firefighters are true heroes as well.

It was required that they take him to the local emergency room first for stabilization, instead of driving the much longer route to TGH. The ER doctors gave him a breathing treatment and did some tests. In collaboration with the transplant team, they called an ICU ambulance to take him back to TGH.

At TGH, the pulmonary doctor was waiting to do an emergency bronchoscopy. This is a procedure done to visualize inside the trachea and lungs. To perform this procedure, a small flexible tube is placed through the nose or mouth. A physician can see the two main air passages of the lungs. Both sputum and tissue biopsy samples are taken. The procedure is short, and lasts between thirty to sixty minutes. This is routinely performed after transplant to look for rejection and infection. In Steve's case, they cleared out mucous in his trachea and lungs. They told us that he developed a large healing mucous scab in the place where his new lungs were attached that started to peel off and blocked his airway. This sudden narrowing of the new airway after the surgery, had never been seen at TGH to cause such severe symptoms like those Steve had experienced. They kept him in the hospital to monitor his condition. After three days, he had no more symptoms and was sent home again.

Since this episode came on suddenly, I was concerned it could have been partially caused by an allergic reaction to our cat. When Steve returned home, after a month away, he sat next to the cat tower covered with all that cat hair and dander. In the past, Steve had experienced occasional mild symptoms of sneezing and itching around cats. So we sent our cat Pippa and the tower on a mini vacation to our friend's house until we were sure it was okay. We cleaned all the carpets and tile.

This time our friends and family joked that maybe Steve could stay home for forty-eight hours. Ironically, exactly two days later, Steve started to experience shortness of breath again after breakfast. We put oxygen on him, and called the transplant team and 911 again. It was the same firefighters who were so helpful the first time. Then it was back to TGH by ambulance for another emergency bronchoscopy. Again they cleared out mucous from his lungs and trachea. This time they kept him in the hospital for eleven more days to figure out what was causing the problem.

Steve and I joked about the fact that on both of those days I had given him peanut butter toast for breakfast. Peanut butter had been one of his favorite foods throughout his entire life. Of course, he jokingly told the doctors that I was trying to kill him. The doctors said it probably had nothing to do with the peanut butter. However, we felt otherwise and vowed that he would not be eating it again anytime soon.

He was already taking meds for gastroesophageal reflux disease (GERD) to protect the new lungs from acid damage. The doctors did a swallow and upper GI study this time. They concluded that his esophagus was having spasms that caused Steve to choke on thick food. They added in an esophageal muscle relaxant to help his esophagus pass food. We were given instructions to stay away from thick food like peanut butter for now.

He was finally released from the hospital again and stayed home for a while. Three months after those episodes, we let our guard down and he ate a peanut butter cookie. Within thirty minutes he started to feel tight in the chest. This time he was able to stay home and breathe through it after talking to the transplant center. It was not as bad of a reaction on this occasion.

The next time we were at the transplant clinic for a follow-up appointment, they ran a blood test to check for peanut allergy. Sure enough, he tested positive. Although they ran many different lab tests routinely after transplant, allergy testing is not one of them. He had apparently acquired this peanut allergy from the donor through his new lungs. Our feeling about peanut butter was then confirmed. It completely surprised the transplant doctors because this situation had never happened at TGH with a lung transplant recipient before.

Due to the serious nature of his reaction, especially related to the lungs and breathing, the hospital is now making a point to inform recipients of donor allergies moving forward. Steve's new nickname from the transplant pulmonologist was "peanut butter boy!" It makes sense that other transplanted organs like kidney or liver should not cause as much of a respiratory allergic reaction due to how they function in the body. The lung transplant programs are newer than other organ programs, so there is still much to learn. As a result of Steve's allergic reaction, the lung donor programs adapted a new protocol to inform the recipient of any allergies.

REVIEW

1. Going home for Steve was short lived due to an unusual allergic reaction in his new lungs to peanuts, which he acquired from the donor.

2. Post-transplant patients have strict monitoring protocols along with dietary guidelines to ensure survival.

3. Donations like food along with emotional support from family and friends were helpful. Don't be afraid to ask for help and be specific about what you need.

Take a Breath

CHAPTER 7: LIFE AFTER LUNG TRANSPLANT

For three months post-surgery, we set up a schedule for family and friends to be at the house with Steve at all times. That is the transplant protocol for the safety of the patient. Patients are also not allowed to drive for a few months because of the surgical scar healing and strong narcotic meds for pain. Steve's care team consisted of local relatives, his brother and sister-in-law, Bob and Lois, my dad, Ed and his partner, Renee, our son John, when he was home from college, and myself. Everyone was very happy that they were not on duty when Steve had his allergic reactions. The first three months after transplant is the most cautionary. My sister Sue, an attorney in Boston, came down to visit and helped care for Steve for a week in the beginning. The two of them with their quick wit often became verbal sparring partners on a mission to zing each other with their sharp tongues. She arrived eager to help yet she immediately announced to Steve, "You are NOT allowed to die on my watch, do you understand? Nobody will believe it was an accident and I will be arrested on murder charges for sure!" Zing! Steve had to laugh at that one but quickly recovered saying, "It just might be worth it!" Zing! "Wait!" she answered, "What am I worried about? Only the good die young so Steve, you're gonna live forever!" At that she blared her iPhone playing Billy Joel's famous song and we laughed and had ourselves a small musical party!

In order to detect any signs of infection or rejection, it is mandatory to follow a standard protocol. Follow-up visits at the transplant clinic occurred weekly for eight weeks, followed by every other week for three months, then once-a-month for the first year. Each time he went to the clinic he had blood drawn, chest x-rays, and pulmonary function tests to look for potential problems. Bronchoscopies were also routinely scheduled approximately one, three, five, seven, nine and twelve months after transplant to look for rejection.

For the first three months, when Steve was out of the house he was instructed to wear a mask, avoid crowds, and anyone who is sick. Children especially carry bacteria and viruses, so avoid kissing them on the lips, and perform frequent hand washing. My work as a pediatrician exposed me to many diseases. I would always change and wash well, after work and before I went into the house. Transplant patients are strictly prohibited to be around anyone for six weeks who received a live viral vaccine like measles, mumps, and rubella (MMR), or chickenpox (varicella). This is because transplant recipients, like cancer patients on chemotherapy, could actually get those diseases from the virus that is in the vaccine. Over the counter meds were cautioned against to protect his kidneys and due to the interactions they might have with his other medicines. Gardening is to be avoided during the first six months following surgery due to fungus in the soil. Swimming is to be avoided in the first six months also due to the potential for contamination.

When he was home, Steve was independently caring for his incision, doing physical therapy, and lung breathing exercises. We were following the strict nutritional recommendations as mentioned previously. He also had to learn how to properly take his daily vitals. This included taking his own blood pressure, body temperature, and a micro spirometer measurement, which is designed to measure lung volume. While taking these vitals, Steve also had to make sure none of them hit the danger zone. These are the measurements that would require an immediate call to his doctor. Symptoms including a temperature above 100.5 degrees, chills, shaking, nausea, vomiting, diarrhea, weakness, or fatigue, just to mention a few, are also necessary to monitor. A lung volume measurement from the micro spirometer that dropped greater than 10% had to be reported immediately.

Steve also filled his large med container each week with the meds he took four times a day. As mentioned previously, these meds were to treat and prevent a variety of conditions and included anti-rejection, antibiotics, anti-viral, anti-fungal, anti-clotting, GERD, anti-spasm of esophagus, constipation, pain from surgery, irregular heart rate, blood pressure, and general vitamins. In the beginning he had to swallow over forty pills a day. The pharmacy co-pay for all these prescribed meds came to over $500 for the first month.

With this extensive and time-consuming protocol, it was helpful that Steve had always been an independent person with a great sense of humor. He continued to retain as much of his independence as possible. He set his iPhone alarm for four different times a day when he needed to take his meds. He told his iPhone to call him "Bubble Boy", which would send us all into hysterical laughter. Bubble Boy was a joke from an episode of Seinfeld, involving a kid who had basically no immune system. The boy lived in a plastic room to avoid germs and was jokingly called Bubble Boy.

Specifically, the anti-rejection meds can weaken and lower the white blood cells, which are needed to fight off infections. Lung transplant recipients have a higher rate of infection in the lungs compared to other types of transplants. This increased rate of infection is thought to be caused by both the direct exposure to inhaled microorganisms and the decreased capacity to cough and clear mucous due to the nerves cut during surgery. This infection risk is greatest in the early post-operative period, when the dosage of immune-suppressive drugs is highest. There are many specific kinds of infections that transplant patients are susceptible to, like bacterial upper and lower respiratory tract infections; viral infections, such as respiratory syncytial virus (RSV); cytomegalovirus (CMV), herpes simplex virus, and fungal infections from yeast or mold.

Although all transplant patients are placed on meds to combat these infections, they are tailored to each patient's needs as time passes. The blood of both donor and recipient is routinely tested for a virus called cytomegalovirus (CMV). CMV is common and can be found in the blood of 50-80% of the general population. It turns out that Steve's donor had this CMV infection in the blood, but Steve's blood tested negative. Since the donor was positive they had to stop the CMV in the transplanted lungs from making Steve's body sick. For three months after the transplant, Steve had to take special IV infusions of antiviral and immunoglobulin meds to treat CMV infection. After those infusions, he was closely monitored for signs of recurrent CMV infection. The symptoms of CMV are usually mild with fever, cough, and fatigue. Many times patients do not realize they are battling this virus. The symptoms in normal patients can be so mild that patients don't seek medical care. They just manage their symptoms at home. For immune-suppressed patients, CMV can cause serious problems, including rejection of the transplanted organ.

Six months following his transplant, Steve got the news regarding his biopsy from his routine bronchoscopy; he needed to come back in for intense IV anti-rejection treatment. He was having no noticeable symptoms. He hadn't felt any different. Surprisingly, it can be difficult to tell if patients are rejecting their newly transplanted lungs. Patients don't always show symptoms of rejection such as shortness of breath, temperatures of 99.6 degrees or greater, chills, fatigue, weakness, general malaise, persistent cough, decreased exercise tolerance, or symptoms similar to a flu or cold.

Once again, Steve was admitted to the transplant floor. A specially trained nurse had to put a central line in him and started a type of med that is made from rabbit serum called thymoglobulin. It's so strong that they had to monitor him closely and could only give him the dosage every other day, as long as his cell counts were okay. When he was getting the thymoglobulin, they kept asking him how he felt. He has such a high tolerance to pain. His answer was always, "I feel fine." He even joked, "except I'm starting to grow pointy ears and a fuzzy tail!"" He stayed in the hospital for a week that time and then was released home. His birthday came and our daughter Megan, a practical joker like her father, had to send him a special birthday package...In it was a large jar of peanut butter! That prank brought a smile to Steve's face.

All along the way, they continued to adjust his meds. The goal was to get Steve off as many as possible. At first, they weaned off his pain meds and anti-clotting meds soon after the surgery. His antibiotics were slowly decreased but he remained on some preventative antibiotics, anti-virals, and anti-fungals. He was being monitored closely for CMV as mentioned earlier. After a year, the doctors were going to stop his anti-viral med but began to notice a drop in his white cell count, a sign of

CMV infection. They noted his blood test for CMV was elevated again. That lead back to an increase in the anti-viral meds and close blood monitoring. In order to boost his white cell count, he received a drug called neupogen as an injection. These treatments helped to get his blood count back on track and he finally beat the CMV.

At eighteen months post-transplant, Steve developed a fever and quickly deteriorated over hours with signs of sepsis. This is a serious and often fatal infection of the blood. Any fever requires a visit to the hospital for evaluation. Steve ended up getting admitted and placed on strong IV antibiotics for a week over Christmas. He didn't even realize that he developed an infected skin spot on his back that turned into an abscess and was spreading into his blood. He tells everyone that he was almost killed by a zit!

Unfortunately, the life-long anti-rejection meds can have serious complications to watch out for including high blood pressure, high cholesterol, and blockage of arteries, which can lead to heart damage, diabetes, cancer, along with liver and kidney damage. Abnormalities such as anemia, osteoporosis, muscle weakness, headaches, tremors, and glaucoma are common problems. Typically, any medical condition present prior to transplant can be enhanced by the meds. For instance, Steve battled with migraine headaches before the transplant. Now as a side effect of the meds, he deals with migraines that induce vomiting and confine him to a dark bedroom for the day.

TGH statistics show the most common lung transplant patient is fifty to sixty-four years of age. Up to 40%

continue to work at least part-time. Most say they have no physical restrictions. At first, Steve began working from home again. Within a few months, he was able to go in part-time with varied hours. This was so helpful because many days he did not feel well enough to go to work.

As you can see from his schedule, life for Steve is far from normal but he is thankful for a second chance at life and for all the assistance his family and friends have given him. He is extremely resilient with a great attitude.

Intimacy can be enjoyed again after transplant. The transplant informational handouts also addressed this issue of sexual activity. It was not too long after he came home, and a good sign that he was on the right track, when Steve was feeling frisky again. I was nervous at first but then pleased to enjoy our intimate relationship like we did before the transplant.

Our relationship has changed and strengthened since his illness. Daily there is a sense that we are in this together as a team. Family and friends are standing behind Steve, supporting his back as he faces the war against pulmonary fibrosis and the recovery from lung transplant. The whole experience of a lung transplant is far more complicated than we could have ever imagined. It is truly an all-encompassing life-long commitment. For survival, we must work together and find ourselves back to our initial relationship where we depend on each other more.

Ironically as I joked before the surgery, it seems as though Steve's personality or attitude has changed about life. In essence he did receive a personality transplant of sorts. Our life has been jolted or interrupted by Steve's sudden and severe illness. We have gotten used to a completely new normal. Caution is required for traveling or situations with crowds of people in order to avoid germs. The protocol for travel is to locate the closest transplant hospital in case Steve experiences problems on vacation. At almost two years later, he has moments that feel parts of life are back to normal. Our children have grown closer to us, also, and stay in touch. We all have a sense that life is fragile and that we must be grateful and present for each moment. Now we all can take a slow, deep, thankful breath.

REVIEW

1. The body will always view the transplanted lungs as foreign and will try to reject the organ, so meds and strict protocols are followed to ensure survival.

2. Lung transplant is quite complicated, and requires a life-long commitment. The anti-rejection meds can have serious side-effects and complications to monitor.

3. The overall survival rate one year post-lung transplant is 80-90% and 40% continue to work at least part-time with no physical restrictions.

4. As a patient, it's especially helpful and empowering to be independent and have a good sense of humor. Life is fragile, be thankful and present for each moment.

Karen A. Kelly M.D.

CHAPTER 8: CHARACTERISTICS FROM THE DONOR

Organ donors can pass much more than a "new life" to the recipient. It is interesting and a little "science fiction-like" to imagine that when someone receives a transplant they acquire all the tissue and DNA of another person. Steve's body has assumed the DNA of his donor from the lung tissue. It is still unknown as to how this incorporated DNA can influence the recipient at the cellular level and beyond. Whether this DNA expresses some characteristics onto the recipient's body remains uncertain.

In Steve's case, he definitely acquired a peanut allergy from the donor. As mentioned earlier, Steve felt that his peanut allergy was getting milder, from his experience with a peanut butter cookie that he had three months after the transplant. He had experienced a much milder reaction then. Nevertheless, he had been very careful about not having peanuts since. Twenty months after receiving his transplant he was leaving work and ate two small pieces of unlabeled chocolate. He thought it tasted minty so he never imagined there were peanuts in it. He started to feel a slight chest tightness as he was driving out of work about an hour later, but thought he was fine. As he sat in traffic on the way home that afternoon, he felt a wave of nausea, diarrhea, and lightheadedness. He realized that he needed to pull over immediately but was unable to get around traffic. He put his car in neutral and immediately passed out.

The nice, young couple in the car ahead, that he rolled into, came out to help him. He proceeded to pass out two more times and was taken to the hospital by ambulance. At the hospital, he experienced forceful vomiting, diarrhea, throat, and facial swelling. As evidenced by this experience, the peanut allergy he received from the donor appeared not to be going away, but actually to be totally incorporated into all the cells of his body including skin, blood, brain, and intestines. His immune system appeared to be changed by the donor. He did get referred to an allergist in order to understand how this can affect him and the transplant. That investigation is still ongoing.

Transplant-acquired allergy was first described after a bone marrow transplant and mostly thought to be transient. Food allergy following organ transplant is thought to be rare, mostly occurring in children. Two cases were described in the past five years in adult women that like Steve, acquired a peanut allergy from their lung donor. Another case was of a woman who initially had a peanut allergy from her lung donor but after a year became completely non-allergic. She had a transient allergic reaction. There are many reports of peanut allergies after liver, kidney, and pancreas transplant providing scientific support to the transfer of some food allergies by transplant.

(ncbi.nlm.nih.gov/pubmed)

There is another described phenomenon called "cell memory theory" where the donor cells retain a "memory" from the transplanted organ that can then transfer characteristics to the recipient like something from a "science fiction" thriller. There are many real life stories of transplanted patients feeling cravings for things that they have never wanted before only to find out that the donor was fond of that particular food. This theory is not thoroughly scientifically validated, but there are stories that seem to confirm that the donor may actually transfer traits like behaviors and emotions to the recipient. These behaviors and emotions acquired by the recipient from the original donor are thought to be due to memories stored in the neurons of the donated organs. Certain types of organs, like the heart, are said to be more susceptible to this "cell memory".

Studies have suggested that large transplanted organs like the heart, liver, and kidneys have neural networks that may act like "little brains" to store memories and characteristics of the donor. There are reports from university research of recipients having changed their preferences for food, music, recreational, and career activities. These changes were actually found to correlate with those of their donor's. In one case of a woman who received a liver transplant, it was found after nine months that her blood type and immune system had changed completely to that of the organ donors. In essence, her liver transplant had also taken over and given her the equivalent of a bone marrow transplant.

Tissues like transplanted corneas do not appear to hold any nerve memory cells. Since the lungs are newer in the organ transplant arena, only time and research will tell us if they also will act like other large organs and transfer "cell memory".

In Steve's case the peanut allergy was definitely transferred from the lungs. Steve had never had any food allergies before the transplant. He doesn't appear to have any other cravings or personal preferences that have changed since the transplant. His personality traits do not appear to be different after the transplant. His attitude has changed in that he is humbled and thankful for receiving a second chance at life.

REVIEW

1. A transplant recipient assumes the DNA of that organ and it is unknown as to how that may affect their body. Steve definitely acquired a life-threatening peanut allergy from his donor.

2. Donors may pass on traits or characteristics to the recipient through a process called "cell memory theory," but this is not scientifically validated.

3. It is believed, but not confirmed, that certain organs like the heart, liver, and kidneys have neural networks that may act like "little brains" and store memories or characteristics of the donor.

4. There are confirmed studies of food allergies being transferred but since lungs are newer to transplant, only time and research will tell us if they can transfer other characteristics to the donor.

Karen A. Kelly M.D.

CHAPTER 9: CAREGIVERS: STOP, LAUGH, AND BREATHE

As a caregiver, experiencing such a serious illness requiring hospitalization, along with providing constant care and support, can put a strain on the people and relationships at home and at work. As Steve's primary caretaker, I was fortunate and thankful to the partners in my group practice for allowing me to easily take time off with him following his surgery. They allowed me to work my schedule around the care team and each member of our family was able to help out in their own way.

My daughter Megan spent time with her Dad before the transplant and then went back to her life in New York City during the weeks he was recovering. She was able to get regular updates and came back to visit frequently throughout his lengthy recovery. This worked out well for her ability to cope with her Dad's serious illness. My son was able to help with his Dad's care on weekends when he was home from college, since he was close by and home often.

We are incredibly thankful for the dedication and support of all the members of Steve's care team, his brother and sister in law, Bob and Lois, my Dad, Renee and my sister Sue. Even our friends, internist Dr. Dave and his wife Leslie, were lifesavers medically and emotionally for us throughout the whole process of Steve's illness, from diagnosis to treatment including emergency situations after the transplant. I am especially appreciative for the assistance given by Dr. Mandel and his wife Karen before the transplant along with Dr Sam. I am also grateful to many people—my partners Drs. Greg, Kathy, Kim, nurse practitioner Linda and my manager Stacy along with my staff, friends, and even my patients and parents—that donated food, time, prayers, and emotional support. All of their help gave us assistance and me much needed breaks.

I went back to work full time after my initial time off with Steve. I was able to also make time for myself by playing tennis, practicing yoga, or just relaxing and reading a book. This time helped me to rejuvenate my energy to be devoted to help Steve with recovery. People at work, both co-workers and parents, would comment to me that they could not believe that I was going through this serious situation with my husband because I looked to have much energy and mental stamina. I was fortunate to have someone like Steve who prides himself in his independence. I believe this attitude significantly helped him rebuild mental and physical strength and speed up his recovery. This upbeat attitude also helped us, his care team, to provide optimal attention to Steve's needs. In fact the nurses at the hospital often complimented him as being an easy to care for patient.

In any given year nearly 29% of the U.S. population or sixty-five million people are caregivers at some point! Caregivers are often the behind the scenes heroes of these medical situations. Many times they provide physical, emotional, and financial support—frequently without any training, and often without recognition or support. They sometimes are sacrificing their own health, both mentally and physically, to take care of their sick loved ones. It is often difficult and, at times unrelenting, dealing with their sick loved one's illness, moods, emotional, and physical needs. This can be a real burden on the caregivers.

Here are some important points to help you, the caregiver:

It is especially important to **STOP** and take care of yourself so that you can be strong and attentive to your sick loved one's needs. The concept is as simple as the instructions on airplanes: "Make sure that you place the oxygen mask over yourself first, so that you can then help your child or loved one." With that same idea in mind, make sure you give yourself the basics like getting rest, eating properly, taking time to exercise, and taking a break from the situation. Caregiving is hard work. It can be emotionally upsetting to watch your loved one going through pain and recovery. Don't ignore your own needs to care for your loved ones. This will ultimately lead to your being unhealthy in mind and body which can limit your ability to provide care. Give yourself credit for doing the best you can. Seek help or emotional support from other caregivers, friends, support groups, or even related websites.

For example, TGH has a nonprofit program called One Breath At A Time, INC (OBAAT) that was established to assist lung transplant recipients and their families with support throughout the process. They provide a temporary home called "Butterfly House" for boarding lung transplant families and patients during all phases of care, initial evaluations, clinic visits, check-ups, and post-op care. TGH also has support groups for caregivers of transplant patients.

Don't be afraid to accept offers of help from friends and family. It is best to be specific about what you need. Do not feel bad about asking for help. Studies show that the giver of help also gets rewarded just as much as the receiver. There are many support programs for caregivers so please take advantage of them, you are actually in essence doing this for your loved one. Remember, by putting on your own breathing mask first, you are better able to help your loved one.

The next piece of advice for caregivers is to advocate and be present as much as you can to speak with the medical personnel about your loved one. Don't be afraid to ask questions and review the medicines. Find a way to communicate with the doctors and nurses. Be open to new ideas and therapies. If that particular doctor is not working well with you, then see if you can consult with another physician in the field. Sometimes another set of eyes seeing the patient's story can be enormously beneficial.

Often another person can communicate in such a way that you understand things better. To help you be an advocate for your loved ones, read about the disease, ask the doctors what you should expect to happen, and become informed. Make sure that the symptoms you are seeing in your loved one match the disease process. You, the caregiver, can monitor them better than anyone else. When the doctor recommends a follow-up appointment, it is assumed that the disease is progressing as expected. If that is not the case, I encourage you to advocate for them by calling to question the medical personnel.

Do not sit around and wait at home for the next scheduled appointment, especially if the condition is getting worse or not following what is expected. Go back to the doctor's office. This could make the difference in uncovering a potential problem early enough to be able to do something about it. This may not make you popular with your loved one or the doctor's office, but you may save your loved one's life or make them more comfortable with their symptoms.

We have all heard the saying "laughter is the best medicine"; in fact studies in the last few decades have shown laughter helps the body in many ways. Laughter has a similar effect as exercise on the body. As we work out and stretch our muscles, this leads to the release of endorphins and a euphoric feeling. Both our pulse and blood pressure goes up and we breathe faster which provides more oxygen to the lungs, which in turn can aid in healing the body. Scientific studies have shown that laughter can improve the body's blood flow, pain tolerance, immune response, blood sugar level, relaxation, and even sleep. There are multiple studies supporting laughter as a healing force. As a caregiver, you could actually provide much needed emotional relief and support by telling a joke or bringing laughter to the medical staff and loved one. It's a joyful feeling when you lighten someone's day and relieve a burden. If you don't know any jokes, just do a little googling. There are lots of "joke-of-the-day" apps and websites for all to enjoy.

There are many wonderful groups of volunteers out there providing caring laughter to patients. One group that I got involved with is called Comedy Connection Caring Clowns who are trained volunteers that bring gentle, appropriate levity and laughter to patients, hospital staff, and nursing homes. Our friends, Dr. Dave and his wife, nurse Leslie, have been involved in a program at Largo Medical Center (LMC) called "Humor 2 You." The program started in 2014 to provide therapeutic humor to patients and their families. The program offers a pleasant diversion from serious situations with gentle gags, magic tricks, jokes, and puppetry. Many times, depending on how serious the situation is, this could be the first time the patient has laughed since being diagnosed.

I actually graduated from "clown college" at LMC in

2014 while Steve was sick. This evening class met once a week and helped me to develop and bring out my inner child or clown. For me, it was a wonderfully silly distraction that helped me to find humor in any situation at home or work. By providing humor to patients, I found myself light hearted with more positive energy. In fact, my clown name is Dr. Lite Heart!

Steve has always been witty with a great sense of humor. He often has a joke or something funny for the doctors or nurses. Dave and Leslie, our friends, brought many practical jokes to the hospital that Steve was happy to play on the medical staff. One joke was a finger that lit up like the pulse-ox machine that monitors the oxygen levels in the blood. It was comical to watch Steve trick the doctor by saying, "Hey Doc, I've been here way too long. Look what's happening to my fingers!" as all of them would light up one at a time. The doctor got a good laugh out of that prank and asked Steve if he could borrow it to play on his other patients and staff. It really helped Steve's spirits and lightened the mood for everyone. For patients and caregivers, humor is a welcome respite from their suffering and isolation, and it has health benefits for all.

Finally, it is also healthy for you the caregiver to take a few moments to breathe deeply. Be totally aware and pay attention to your breathing for short periods. This could be anytime that you can take a few moments for yourself, like in the car driving to the hospital, before you walk in the room, or even while sitting on the toilet. This mindful breathing can be a form of meditation.

The definition of meditation is a narrowing of the

focus that shuts out the external world with a stillness of the body. Even for just a few moments, meditation has been shown to have health benefits including lowering blood pressure, raising the immune system, and improving the ability to concentrate.

What really helped me to be calm and attentive to Steve everyday was that I would listen to calming meditation programs in the car on the way to the hospital. This would allow me to take deep breaths and just concentrate on driving and breathing. Obviously, I did not close my eyes while I was driving, but just the awareness of my breathing provided peace and stress relief. When I got to the hospital, I was calm and centered. I truly feel that practice of awake meditation saved my sanity throughout Steve's illness and hospitalizations. I continue to make time for meditation. I am convinced of the many benefits that it has in my life.

REVIEW

1. Caregivers: take care of yourself with basic needs like rest, nutrition, and exercise, along with breaks away in order to be attentive to your loved one's needs.

2. Be an advocate for your loved one by reading about the disease process, and don't be afraid to ask questions and call or return to the doctor if symptoms are not progressing as expected.

3. Laughter is truly therapeutic to patients, staff, and caregivers, so tell a joke.

4. Take deep breaths or meditate periodically during your day to calm your body and mind.

Karen A. Kelly M.D.

FINAL THOUGHTS

Few sensations are as frightening as not being able to catch your breath. Healthy people may experience shortness of breath in extreme temperatures or after exercise, or even at high altitudes. Persistent or long lasting shortness of breath should be a red flag. If you or a loved one are consistently out of breath, or are making a wheezing or high-pitched sound while breathing that only gets worse with simple activities like walking, then go to a medical doctor.

Before I studied medicine and became a doctor, I believed that medical diagnosis was like a math problem. If I took all the symptoms of a patient's disease and put them together, I could come up with an exact diagnosis and treatment like a math solution. I was really good at math so I thought medicine would be a natural for me.

However, what I've learned from practicing medicine as a pediatrician is that the medical diagnostic process in patients is not straight forward at all. Many times the same symptoms in patients do not equal the same diagnosis or disease. Even the same disease in individual patients can progress differently or even respond differently to the same medical treatment.

This atypical response can be a clue that the diagnosis is changing or incorrect. It could be from the patient not taking the medicines correctly or even at all. Each case presentation can be so unique and different that medical diagnosis is a real art and takes years of practice. Due to the many different disease presentations and symptoms, it is not at all like a math problem that ends with the same solution. In a sense, it's like being a detective and continually uncovering clues to help formulate what disease process is affecting the patient.

In Steve's case, when he was first diagnosed with COPD, we had a clue that something was off by the rapid decline in his condition and his lack of response to the meds initially prescribed to him. We trusted that the doctors were making the best decision at the time. When we informed them that his condition was getting worse, we all realized that something wasn't right. They moved up his visit and changed their medical approach.

There is a lesson to be learned from Steve's story in navigating through the medical maze and advocating for your sick loved one. Because medical diagnosis is not straight forward, even the best doctors can be thrown off by the symptoms and tests. The medical personnel are doing the best they can with the information provided at that time about the patient. The clues or symptoms can change. These changes can provide doctors with hints as to a different diagnosis or treatment. Many times I hear people say that they go to the doctor and nothing was done. Doctors are actually taking another look at the patients' symptoms and clues to the diagnosis. With that information, do your best to work as a team with your doctor. Don't hold back information from your doctor. Many times you may not understand the significance of your symptoms that could be a clue to your doctor. Even if your loved one is not getting better or you feel like you have hit a concrete wall—don't give up. Keep on asking questions and telling people your story. This will many times open an unknown door to new opportunities.

As mentioned earlier, Steve initially did not meet the criteria to be evaluated at the transplant program. We were discouraged and thought that we had to find another option. Miraculously, we were able to get the doctors at the transplant program to look at Steve's CT scan, because of a call from a colleague and friend in the medical field. After reviewing his markedly abnormal scan, they were impressed and changed his diagnosis to idiopathic pulmonary fibrosis, which qualified him to be evaluated by the specialist team. The transplant team realized that other appropriate patients could be missed. After Steve's case, they decided to look at all abnormal CT scans or MRIs of referred patients that didn't meet the criteria for evaluation. The pulmonary doctors would be looking directly at the pictures of the lungs and confirm or amend the diagnosis when appropriate. They realized the diagnosis of idiopathic pulmonary fibrosis and other rare lung diseases are not common which makes them harder to diagnose. In doing this, the transplant team hoped not to overlook any patients who deserve a work-up and consideration for transplant. This change in evaluation saved Steve's life and potentially others' who previously did not qualify.

The diagnosis of irreversible lung disease, like pulmonary fibrosis, is overwhelming and frightening. Steve felt robbed of his physical abilities and future life. Yet, he maintained a great attitude and was positive he would get through it. Watching your loved one deteriorate from this disease is terrifying and stressful for the caregiver. Caregivers need to take care of themselves in order to be there for their loved one. That includes exercise, time to yourself and laughter, laughter, laughter. Getting to the right place for Steve's diagnosis was reassuring. Being told that your husband needs a lung transplant was like being hit with a brick.

Accepting this fact and jumping through all the hoops in order to get on the transplant list was like a medical scavenger hunt in a bad reality TV show. For Steve, going downhill quickly after being put on the transplant list and being admitted to TGH until he got a transplant was devastating and depressing at times. Thanks to the generosity of the donor and family a perfectly matched set of lungs became available for Steve after a few weeks on the list. Watching him recover from the major surgery of the lung transplant with all the tubes and drains went by quickly. Taking deep breaths and calming my breathing every day before going into the hospital was rejuvinating for me. Our experience of coming home and being rushed back by ambulance because of an allergic reaction to peanut butter twice was unbelievable. For Steve, those episodes made him feel fearful and powerless. During his perilous post-transplant journey, he had many major setbacks including rejection, infection, allergic reactions and migraines. Each event and readmission to the hospital chipped away at his confidence level for recovery and was a reality check for him in how he chooses to live his life. Each time he thought, "I should have enjoyed myself more and eaten more ice cream!"

Finally almost two years later, Steve is starting to see a light at the end of the long dark tunnel of his illness. Many days he feels almost back to himself. As mentioned previously, he is working part-time. He is looking forward to a future and setting small goals in order to feel good for three months straight without any health problems. He is confident that his good health will extend to six months and then for an entire year. His life and health responsibilities are complicated and forever changed. He knows he has to be cautious about the risks he chooses to take with exposure to potential diseases or germs. He must take every small problem as potentially life-threatening. Even the common cold in transplant patients can be serious and take weeks to fight off. He is especially thankful and enjoying precious time with his family and friends. But he hasn't forgotten the nurse's warning, "Many people start to feel better, and stop taking their medicine...and then they die."

It is truly a miracle that Steve is still on this earth teasing others and telling jokes with another person's lungs working inside of him. Attitude clearly matters in fighting for your life in any disease. Humor is a welcome relief for suffering patients and has health benefits for all. People like Steve with a positive, independent attitude, a strong will, a purpose for living, and a commitment to struggle will have a better experience. Any patient with an active response to helping their own treatment, rather than a passive acceptance of anything the medical personnel say, will definitely live a longer and more empowered life. The strong stubborn will of the Irish is a blessing for survival but a curse to deal with for caregivers. Caregivers who also stop to take care of themselves, laugh, meditate, advocate and be present for their loved ones will have better success.

Transplant surgery is a modern miracle. The process of getting a transplant is fascinating and complicated for both patients and caregivers. Since 1988 in the United States over 650,000 transplants have occurred! Presently in the United States there are more than 120,000 people on organ transplant waiting lists. Each day an average of over seventy-five people receive an organ transplant. However mostly due to the shortage of organs, over twenty patients die each day waiting for transplants.

Lung transplant is used to treat irreversible diseases like pulmonary fibrosis, COPD, cystic fibrosis and pulmonary hypertension. The lung transplant program at TGH was only ten years old in the summer of 2014. At that time, they had just passed four hundred total lung transplants. Steve is #403. TGH had previously done thirty seven lung transplants in one year from June 2014-15. During that same time period there were 1,700 people listed on the lung transplant waiting lists in the U.S.

Please consider becoming an organ donor. Organ donation can help make sense of tragedy. Many religions believe and encourage organ donation. Our catholic church bulletin had an excerpt from Pope John Paul II which said that donations of organs done in an ethically acceptable manner is a form of heroism and can offer health and even life to the sick who often have no hope.

One organ donor can help many individuals.

To register to be a donor visit:

www.DonateLifeFlorida.org

www.donatelife.net

www.organdonor.gov

You can be a hero and save a life!

Please consider a donation to the LifeLink Legacy Fund to support the LifeLink Foundation's efforts in organ and tissue donation and transplantation.

Please consider a donation to Tampa's non-profit organization for lung transplant patients and families in need called OBAAT (One Breath At A Time), OBAAT.org

Now take a moment again to consciously breathe. Take a breath in and out and appreciate the miracle of your working lungs.

Pictures of Steve:

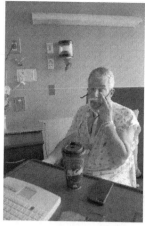

On the 30 liters of oxygen before the transplant being a joker showing his middle finger!

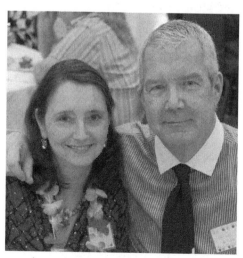

Steve and I at the transplant Christmas party four months after his transplant!

REFERENCES

www.LifeLinkfoundation.org

www. donatelife.net

www.organdonor.gov

www.unos.org

www.lungtxp.com

www.webmd.com

www.webmd.com/balance/features/give-your-body-boost-with-laughter?

www.lungtransplantfoundation.org

www.wikipedia.org

www.SCRTR.org (Scientific Registry of Transplant)

americantransplantfoundation.org

www.rimed.org,Rhode Island Med VOLUME 94 NO. 2 FEBRUARY 2011 Caregiving

www.caregiver.org

www.caregiveraction.org

www.thefreedictionary.com/respirationnhlbi.nih.gov/health/health-topics

www.thoracic.org (COPD)

www.medicaldaily.com/can-organ-transplant-change-recipients-personality-cell-memory-theory-affirms-yes-247498

www.TheComedyConnection.org

www.H2U.com/H2Umagazine

www.cancerguide.org/median_not_msg.html

www.ncbi.nlm.nih.gov/pubmed/22172896/

Karen A. Kelly M.D.

ABOUT THE AUTHOR

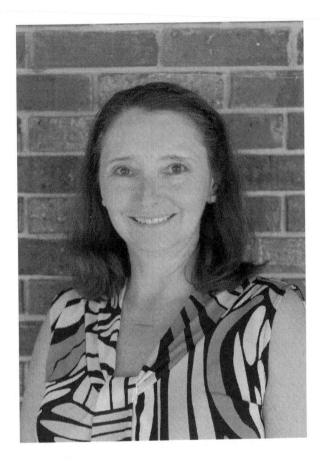

Dr. Karen A. Kelly M.D. is a busy pediatrician practicing for over twenty years in her co-owned group practice Myrtle Ave Pediatrics located in the Tampa Bay area. She absolutely loves her work, along with her patients, their families, and the staff in her practice. She is originally from New England and is a die-hard Patriots and

Red Sox fan. She earned her pre-med undergraduate degree at Northeastern University in Boston, MA, and her medical degree at the University of Mass Medical School in Worcester, MA. Then after deciding to move to the sun, she completed a three-year residency in pediatrics at All Children's Hospital in St. Petersburg, Florida. She served for two years after residency with the National Health Service Program in St Petersburg, Florida practicing in a poor, underserved population.

She married her husband Steve during medical school. They have been married for twenty-five years. They presently live in a quaint town west of Tampa, Dunedin. Steve, the subject of this book, works for Community Health Centers of Pinellas. They have two grown children, Megan and John. Megan graduated from Boston University and is working in New York City in TV production. John is beginning his fourth year in college at USF, Tampa, studying Biology and Computer Science. Her loving family enjoys time together boating, playing cards, and traveling. She has four close siblings who lost their mother to a devastating lung disease in 2001. She is close to her Dad and his partner, Renee, who are snowbirds and live in Clearwater, FL for most of the year.

She is a long term member of the American Academy of Pediatrics, since 1991. Dr. Kelly served as the chairman of pediatrics and the director of the newborn hearing program at Morton Plant Hospital from 2008 to 2012. She serves on the Pinellas immunization team (PITCH) and the tobacco-free coalition of Pinellas committees. She graduated from clown college at Largo Medical Center in 2014 and enjoys performing as Dr. Lite Heart, the caring clown, providing laughter for patients. She loves to use her corny jokes and gags to help her pediatric patients feel at ease in her office. She enjoys playing tennis, practicing yoga, meditating, and reading. This is her first book.

Please feel free to contact her at her practice website: www.Happykidsmd.com or email:kelly.md@verizon.net or visit lungtransplantjourney.com

To learn about Caring Clowns visit:
www.thecomedyconnection.org